MW01292304

HOLD

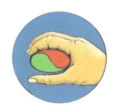

A Chiropractic Examination Aid Using
Muscle Testing

By

Dr. Bruce Vaughan DC, FICC

ISBN 10 1508560293
ISBN 13 9781508560296

I want to acknowledge the assistance and encouragement from my practice colleagues, especially Drs. Alex Pak and Michelle Zhou Mc Culloch, for their help in proof reading and commenting on the manuscript.

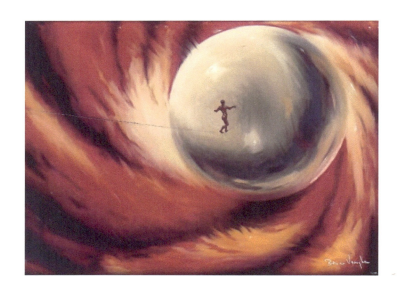

Man's struggle for Homeostasis, by Bruce Vaughan

Table of Contents

INTRODUCTION

Make no mistake, I am not claiming to have invented muscle testing, nor to have improved on it. Muscle testing goes back at least to the 1930s, when two physiotherapists named Kendall, (husband and wife), were working together with Dr. Lovett, an orthopedic surgeon, on polio victims. Their emphasis is on evaluating individual muscle strength to detect weakness and to monitor progress during rehabilitation. Dr. De Jarnette DC started to use some form of muscle testing in his Sacral Occipital Techniques (SOT) as a way to detect neuro-physical dysfunction as it applies to chiropractic. Dr. Goodheart DC made the greatest contribution with Applied Kinesiology (AK).

There are many disciplines that are using some form of mind/body muscle testing, but in this book I am staying with the more physical uses, relating to the diagnosis of neuro-musculo-skeletal problems commonly seen in chiropractic practice.

Some practitioners are unwilling to try muscle testing as they see it as some strange form of witchcraft, voodoo or at least too esoteric for them. It is in fact a very useful and time tested diagnostic adjunct that can, with experience, be an important addition to the routine chiropractic and orthopedic testing protocol.

The following tests are a variety of body/mind tests.

The art of muscle testing — and it is an art — comes from experience. As with so many techniques, it is like learning to ride a bicycle; the theory and science of balancing a bicycle do not prepare you for the day when you go for the first ride. You have to do it, wobbling and falling occasionally until it comes naturally and then away you go.

The series of muscle tests that I describe in this book take but a few seconds, once you are proficient, and they can tell you so much useful information about your patient.

These tests are not a substitute for clinical diligence in chiropractic practice, but an additional tool in the toolbox. As with all tests, you should never rely entirely on one finding, but you should use muscle testing as a pointer, along with other clinical means to reach a diagnosis.

The beginner in muscle testing must be aware of factors that can cloud the outcome. These factors may come from tester/doctor or the testee/patient. The doctor should approach each test with a neutral mind: for example, he may have reached a conclusion from the case history that the patient has a particular problem. By projecting that thought into the test he can sub-consciously influence the outcome. A patient may have a dental malocclusion which when he bites can cause a muscle to weaken, in such a case the doctor must ask the patient to relax his jaw during the test. The patient may have a shoulder problem, which is why the arm should be tested before making a contact.

The muscle tests are means of seeking the truth and the body does not lie: as a test of this, ask someone to tell you either his real name, or a false name and then test for muscle strength, if the person lies and gives a name that is not his the muscle will weaken: try it. Who needs sophisticated lie detectors when you have muscle testing?

The tests are divided into 'standing tests' that take just about twenty seconds and then either one set of 'prone tests' again around twenty seconds, or a set of 'supine tests', even shorter, according to the outcome of the 'standing tests'.
I have included a few other tests that I have found useful and I hope that you will too.

For these tests to become a routine part of your examination I suggest you do as I do and do them with every patient on every visit; things change between visits and these simple tests can keep you current.

For the maintenance or wellness patient the few seconds spent doing the muscle tests can warn you of potential problems that need your attention.

Muscle tests are not technique specific, by this I mean that they be used to help you come to a diagnosis and check for progress, whatever your preferred approach to chiropractic.

If you are new to this testing approach, please take the time to perfect the tests before you start testing your patients. It is important for you to be confident and competent in this approach, so that the patient has the same confidence in your competence. Your hesitation or doubt will be transmitted to the patient, making the outcome equally doubtful; don't lose heart if it does not seem to work at first. It takes time to get the feel for the weak arm. You should not over-power the patient; the whole test is in the first response.

I suggest that you practice on colleagues or family, so that you can detect the subtle difference between a strong, immediate response and a weak, delayed or mushy one. What do I mean by mushy? A normal response should be immediate, so that you feel the solid resistance to your pressure. A patient may sometimes be able to resist you, even when there is a 'weak' response, but there is a slight delay. It is as if the body is prepared for the downward force of your hand based on the learned response from the 'normal' responses, but has to adjust the response when the test challenge creates a 'weak' arm. This adjustment takes a very short time, but it is detectible.

It is quite common for the 'weak' arm to just give way, often surprising the patient. When done correctly it is a very convincing phenomenon and one that the patient looks for on future visits.

To practice on colleagues or family, you can use the true or false questions, I mentioned above, to get the feel of the 'normal' or 'weak' responses. First brief them that you are going to ask them questions and you want them to either tell the truth or lie. The body does not accept a lie and the arm will go weak when the person tells a lie.

Once you have the feeling of a 'weak' muscle, then start practicing on the various points for testing. Do it on colleagues for a while until you feel confident.

I am sure that you will find these tests useful once you are ready to do them as I do, on every patient every visit.

THE FIVE STANDING TESTS.

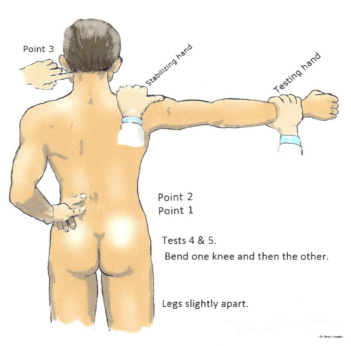

Point 3

Stabilizing hand

Testing hand

Point 2
Point 1

Tests 4 & 5.
Bend one knee and then the other.

Legs slightly apart.

These five tests are designed to identify possible problems in the low back and pelvis. They take just a few seconds and can give you some useful information.

You start by asking the patient to stand in front of you, facing away from you, the patient's feet should be apart by about nine to twelve inches with equal weight on each foot.

Now ask the patient to raise one arm out to the side so that it is horizontal to the floor — I personally prefer the right arm, but that is just because it fits my examining space and my being left handed may have something to do with it — it doesn't matter which hand you use in most cases.

The exception is when testing the styloid process; according to Dr. De Jarnette the left styloid process apparently indicates a disc problem. This is another reason for me to use the right hand for testing and the left for placement.

Explain that you are going to put a downward pressure on the extended arm when you say "hold" and you want the patient to resist with an equal amount of strength, tell him/her it is not a contest.

A positive response is an immediate strong reaction, whereas a negative one feels mushy, as if there is a delayed response. It is the immediate response that matters, not the strength. It is not a competition; a body builder can recover quickly and over power you, but the initial hesitation has already told you what you want to know.

Say "hold" and apply a quick downward force, just enough to feel a positive and immediate response.

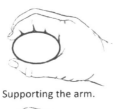

Supporting the arm.

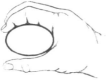

Testing.

As you apply pressure open the hand so that the pressure is on the upper surface of the patient's arm, so that the arm is free to follow its natural arc with the downward pressure.

Continuing to grip the wrist whilst pushing the arm down can cause discomfort for the patient and thus give a false result. This is really only relevant if the arm collapses with the pressure.

STANDING TEST ONE:

Looking for an ilio-sacral jamming problem (CAT I in SOT).

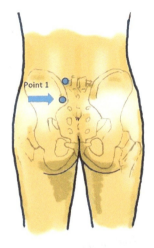

Take the patient's other hand and position the thumb on the posterior superior spine of the iliac crest (PSIS). Just a contact is enough; this is a localization test rather than a challenge test.

Once again say "hold" and exert the same amount of pressure to the extended arm. Did it go weak? Or did it stay strong? Weakness can be merely a slightly mushy or delayed response, or a definite drop of the arm; once you detect either a positive response or weaker or mushy response there is no need to press the arm any further; pushing hard down on a weakened arm can harm it.

A weak response indicates an ilio-sacral locking, (PI/AS) restricting the normal but slight motion between the sacrum and the ilia on either side. It is a jammed pelvis causing a lack of respiratory motion which a vital part of the cerebro-spinal fluid pump mechanism.

Look for a forward and backward sway to confirm this. This is the body's method of compensating for a compromised CSF pump.

STANDING TEST TWO:

Looking for a weakness in the Sacro-iliac joint (CAT II)

Move the thumb to a point just medial to the iliac crest and lateral to the spinous process of L5; there is little fleshy spot there.

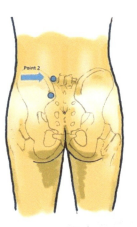

Again say "hold" etc, you know the drill now.

This is also a localization test, so all that is required is a contact, without exerting pressure.

A weak or mushy arm will indicate a Sacro-iliac sprain/strain or rarely a separation.

The all-important weight-bearing function of the Sacro-iliac is impaired.

STANDING TEST THREE:

Looking for signs of a disc involvement.

Bring the patient's index finger up to a point an inch or so below the mastoid process to contact the left styloid process at the point where it joins the Hyoid ligament; easy does it, this a sensitive area.

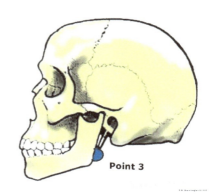

Point 3

Again say "hold" etc.

This is also a localization test which indicates a connective tissue involvement and so points to a possible disc involvement.

Dr. De Jarnette theorizes that the left styloid process should be tested for disc involvement, as I mentioned earlier, this is one reason why I make a habit of using the right arm for testing and the left arm for contact.

If positive for a disc, then palpation of the two styloids can show laterality of the bulge. A sensitive styloid indicates an ipsilateral bulge.

STANDING TESTS FOUR AND FIVE:

These are looking for functional problems in the lower lumbar spine and the pelvis.

Ask the patient to drop his placing hand to his side and then bend one knee slightly, keeping the heel on the ground. Test, then ask him/her to straighten that leg and bend the other one and test again. If one or the other goes weak the prone tests will isolate the particular problem.

I see these two tests as part of one because by changing from one bent leg to another the low back and pelvis are mechanically challenged.

These are functional challenge tests.

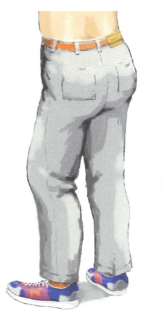

The heel stays on the ground.

As the patient changes weight from one side to another it challenges the lumbo-sacral dynamics as well as the pelvis' ability to adapt to the change.

The specific problem can then be found in the Prone tests.

TIMING FOR STANDING TESTS.

Just how long is this set of tests going to take you, once you are familiar with the routine?

Let's time it. Read the following, whilst imagining yourself doing the action:

Ask the patient to stand facing away from you, with the testing arm outstretched and feet apart by about nine to ten inches.

Test the arm.
Place contact thumb on point 1.
Say hold. Test arm.
Place contact thumb on point 2.
Say hold. Test arm.
Place contact finger on point 3.
Say hold. Test arm.

Patient bends one knee.

Say hold. Test arm.

Patient bends other knee.

Say hold. Test arm.

The whole standing routine takes just as long as it took for you to read the above list; about <u>twenty to thirty seconds</u>.

It will be a little longer for the first time the patient has done it, because you have to explain things, but not much longer.

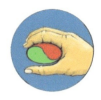

PRONE TESTING.

With the patient lying prone, get him/her to extend one arm at right angles to the body and level to the floor (most people have a preferred side to operate from, so make that the testing side).

Test for a strong arm, if the arm is weak for some reason, for example: the patient may have a shoulder problem, then go to the opposite side and work from there.

To test, contact the patient's wrist and as you say 'hold' apply force, opening the hand slightly so that you are only contacting the upper part of the wrist

PRONE TESTS 1 and 2
(PSIS on both sides)

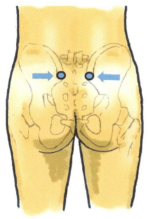

The doctor puts a downward pressure (P to A) on one Posterior superior iliac spine, (PSIS) and test (Say "hold" and press), then goes to the opposite PSIS and tests.

This is a challenge test, but it does not need heavy pressure.

By slightly forcing the PSIS Anterior you are worsening the AS condition, causing the arm to go weak.

A weakness will indicate that the PSIS on that side has moved Anterior and Superior (AS).

PRONE TESTS 3 and 4

(Ischia on both sides.)

The doctor puts a downward (P to A) pressure on the ischial tuberosity, first one side and test, then the other and again test.

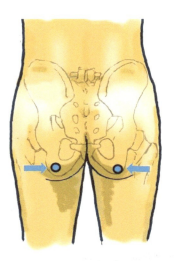

A weak muscle will indicate that the Ischium is Anterior, therefore the PSIS is Posterior Inferior (PI) on that side.

You may well find that the weak side in these tests is on the opposite side to the prone test 1 or 2 weakness.

I always do a leg check whether there is a positive sign in the above four tests, or not.

PRONE TESTS 5 and 6
(Base of the sacrum.)

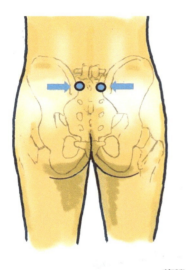

Put a downward pressure (A to P) on one side of the base of the sacrum and then the other side.

A weakness indicates a rotation of the sacrum within the pelvis on that side.

This may be a jamming rotation that does not destabilize the SI joint.

PRONE TESTS 7 and 8
(Apex of the sacrum.)

Exert a pressure A to P on one side of the sacral apex and then the other. A weakness will indicate a twist within the sacrum itself.

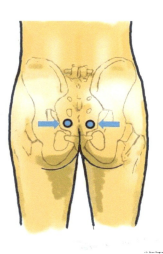

The Apex has twisted away from the contact point, ie anterior; the side to adjust would be the opposite side which will have gone posterior.

This can occur if a patient has bumped against something and caused a jarring of the sacral apex.

I have quite often found that pain within the pelvis that does not respond to other pelvic or lumbar adjustments can be caused by a twist within the sacrum.

Remember that the living sacrum is not fused as a solid block and there is subtle movement between the individual segments. The first three segments are held by the Ilio-sacral articulations, but the apex is vulnerable to impact and can get subluxated.

PRONE TESTS 9 and 10.
(Ilio-sacral sheer.)

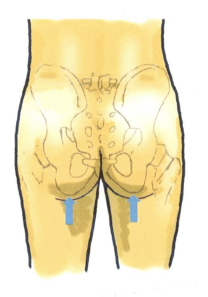

When there is a pelvic pain that does not seem to be resolved with normal low back/pelvic routine adjusting.

Exert a Cephalic (towards the head) pressure to the under surface of one ischium and then the other.

A weakness shows that there is a sheer displacement between the sacrum and the ilia.

The Ilia has gone superior or the sacrum has gone inferior (six of one half a dozen of the other). The adjustment would be on the lateral margin of the Sacrum, on the same side forcing it superior.

This injury can occur, for instance, if a person steps off a step awkwardly; perhaps when he miscalculates the height of a step or does not see a curb coming, especially if he lands with a straight leg.

PRONE TESTS 11 and 12.
(5th lumber rotation.)

Press against the lateral margin of the spinous process of the 5th lumbar vertebra, left to right first and then right to left.

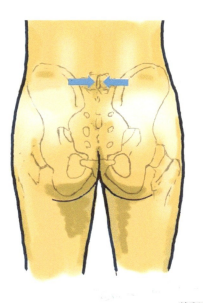

Weakness indicates a probable rotation of L5 away from the direction of pressure, as indicated.

This is a challenge test. By putting pressure against the spinous process you are aggravating the condition.

Note: the same techniques can be used on other segments of the spine.

OPTIONAL TEST FOR 5th LUMBAR POSTERIORITY.

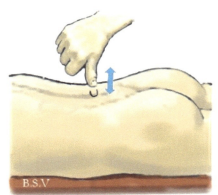

A direct downward (A to P) bounce applied directly onto the spinous process of L5.

This requires a quick push and an even quicker withdrawal, before reaching the point of full resistance.

By this I mean before the point when the posterior joints are fully compressed by the pressure.

A weakness shows that the L5 is directly posterior.

When the vertebra is pushed forward, followed by a quick withdrawal, the rebound forces the vertebra posterior, thus aggravating the posterior displacement.

Note: You should rule out a possible spondylolisthesis first.

TIMING FOR PRONE TESTS.

Let's time this set of prone tests.

The patient is lying prone. Ask the patient to extend the testing arm out to the side. Test the arm.
Dr. places his thumb on point 1.
Say 'hold' and test arm.
Dr. places his thumb on point 2
Say 'hold' and test arm.
Dr. places his thumb on point 3
Say 'hold' and test arm.
Dr. places his thumb on point 4
Say 'hold' and test arm.
Dr. places his thumb on point 5
Say 'hold' and test arm.
Dr. places his thumb on point 6
Say 'hold' and test arm.
Dr. places his thumb on point 7
Say 'hold' and test arm.
Dr. places his thumb on point 8
Say 'hold' and test arm.
Dr. places his thumb on point 9
Say 'hold' and test arm.
Dr. places his thumb on point 10
Say 'hold' and test arm.
Dr. places his thumb on point 11
Say 'hold' and test arm.
Dr. places his thumb on point 12
Say 'hold' and test arm.
And you are done.

Again this takes as long as it takes to read whilst visualizing the above list. <u>Between twenty and thirty seconds</u> or so.

As it is the doctor who is moving from one point to another, there is little explanation required, all the patient has to do is respond to the command 'HOLD', so the whole set of tests can be done quite quickly.

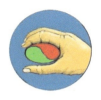

SUPINE TESTING.

These tests are indicated when the Standing Test 2 went weak.

This indicates a sprain/strain/separation of the sacro-iliac. Cat II in SOT lingo.

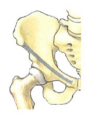 You are testing the upper and lower fossa of the sacro-iliac joint. The test area is the Inguinal (Poupart's) Ligament.

With the patient lying supine, the doctor stands adjacent to the patient's mid-thigh facing towards the patient's opposite shoulder.

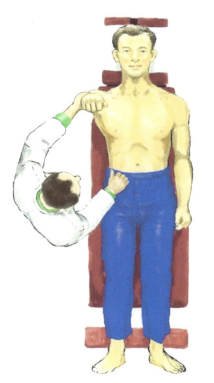

Ask him/her to raise the arm closest to you directly perpendicular and to resist when you say "hold", at which point you exert a test pressure towards the feet (Caudal).

Just as before, you are looking for an immediate response rather than a weak, mushy or delayed response. You should be aware of the immediate response; it does not take a full downward swing to detect a weak arm.

It is not a competition.

As you exert pressure open the hand so that you are only contacting the upper surface of the patient's wrist.

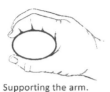
Supporting the arm.

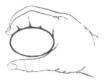
Testing.

A reminder.

As the arm is pressed in each of the testing positions it describes an arc, so that a firm grip around the wrist would cause discomfort if the arm collapses, as it sometimes does.

THE SUPINE TEST.

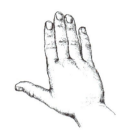

To find the first test point, the Anterior Superior Iliac Spine (ASIS), use a flat hand (See the Glass Hand description below*), fingers firmly straight, and press down where you believe that the ASIS should be. As a chiropractor you should have acquired a sensitivity for all types of palpation.

The moment you feel the boney protuberance under your hand mark that point visually as if you are seeing it through your hand, whilst keeping your eye on that point; cup the hand so that all four fingertips are level, and contact the ASIS protuberance with the index

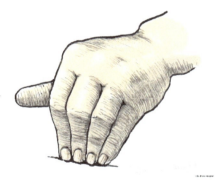

finger and then slide all four fingers medially until they are all on the lateral half of the inguinal ligament.

Say "hold" as you simultaneously press the lateral (upper) half of the inguinal ligament and test the arm. The pressure should be no more than you could take on your own eyeball.

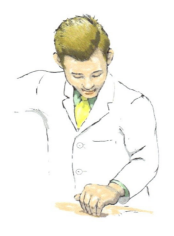

Then slide the four fingers medially along the inguinal ligament (remember that the inguinal ligament describes a shallow arc) until the little finger feels the pubis, then back off until you are on the medial (lower) half of the ligament and repeat the test.

Change sides and repeat the whole test from the opposite side of the patient.

A weakness at a point confirms the standing test, ie: there is a sacro-iliac sprain/strain or separation involvement.

The doctor should now check for a short or long leg on the side of weakness. Notice if the leg is short on the same side as the upper fossa weakness (the first point tested on each side), or long on the side of the lower fossa weakness, then we are ready to adjust (Block in SOT protocol).

If the leg lengths do not check out correctly, then look for other problems such as the Psoas, Diaphragm or Upper Cervicals.

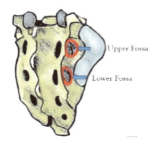

The upper (lateral) half of the Inguinal ligament reflects the status of the Upper Foss of the Sacrum, and the lower (medial) half reflects the status of the Lower Fossa of the Sacrum.

34

The Glass Hand.

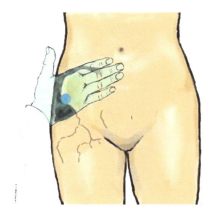

To use the 'glass hand' place the locating hand an inch or so above the point where you believe that the ASIS is situated. The hand should be rigid, completely flat; now lower it to the point until you just feel the bony prominence (ASIS) under the hand.

There is no need to press any further, just be aware of the hard surface below your hand. Do not curl the fingers. Imagine that the hand is made of glass and you can see through it to the point of contact.

Keep your eye on that point as you withdraw the hand and position the fingers in preparation to contact the ASIS with the index finger and then slide all four fingers medially onto the lateral half of the inguinal ligament (Poupart's ligament).

These tests are localization tests that are looking for a weakness in the important weight-bearing articulation of the SI joint.

The Hyaline Cartilage becomes wet and mobile allowing for a debilitating shift in the articulation. Normally there is only a very subtle movement in the SI joint.

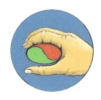

A SUMMARY OF THE TESTING PROTOCOL.

Once you have mastered this set of tests, you will find that they can be done quickly during routine visits. The information they give you can be put to immediate use. Remember that the muscle tests that I have described should not be seen as definitive diagnoses, but recognized as indicators that can point the way to a differential diagnosis when confirmed by case history and other tests where indicated. So what do they indicate?

The standing tests give us four main areas of concern.

Standing Test One, shows a pelvic distortion/jamming (PI/AS). Adjustments vary according to technic used, Gonstead side posture, Thompson drop, SOT blocking etc.

The PRONE tests follow any weakness seen here.

Standing Test Two, Is specific for a Ilio-sacral weakness. Again use your own technic for adjustment. I personally prefer the SOT blocking for this, as it is a problem of too much motion in the S/I and so manipulation would tend to further the unwanted mobility.

The SUPINE tests follow if there is a weakness.

Standing Test Three, indicates a possible disc problem and should be seen as a Red Flag. Do whatever further tests necessary to make sure that your Tx is appropriate. This can vary from manual adjustments, Flexion-extension, SOT blocking, etc, or ultimately surgery. Proceed with caution.

The PRONE tests follow where there is a weakness.

Standing Tests Four and Five, indicate a dynamic problem in the lumbo-pelvic area. These are amenable to adjustments, using the technic of your choice.

The PRONE tests follow where indicated.

The prone tests cover all the standing test weaknesses except that of Test Two.

Prone tests one and two, look an AS on one side or another.

Prone tests three and four, look for a PI on one side or the other.

Prone tests five and six, look for a sacral rotation within the pelvis.

Prone tests seven and eight, look for a rotation within the sacrum itself.

Prone tests nine and ten, look for a sheer (sliding) jamming between the sacrum and the ilia.

Prone tests eleven and twelve, look for rotation of L5. The rotation is away from the direction of contact.

THE SUPINE TESTS, are specific to the weakness in the weight-bearing articulation of the sacro-iliac. Again use your own method of addressing this problem. As I mentioned earlier, I prefer the SOT blocking for this particular problem as it is non-invasive and restores the correct positioning without creating more unwanted mobility in the joints.

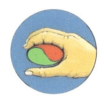

SURROGATE TESTING.

For a variety of reasons it may not be possible to get the patient to cooperate during the testing process. Reasons can vary from being too young, mentally challenged or too frail.

There are various ways to meet this challenge.

1. Use someone else to be a surrogate test subject. Where possible this should be a relative or care giver. The doctor touches the points and instead of testing the patient's arm, the doctor tests the surrogate's arm in the same way that he would have tested the patient.

   The difference here is the fact that the doctor cannot stabilize the patient's shoulder while testing, so make sure that the pressure each time is directly towards the floor.

   This sounds a bit weird at first, but it does work and can be a useful tool where needed.

   Opinions vary as to whether the patient should be in contact with the patient. It does not appear to make a difference. It is mind-body to mind-body connection, rather than a direct body to body connection that seems to be important.

Certainly a mother can hold her baby while you test the baby through the mother.

2. Where a patient is unable to reach the points in the standing tests, due to shoulder injury or other weakness, the doctor can contact the test points.

3. Care should be taken, as with the surrogate test in #1 above, to not destabilize the patient due to the lack of a stabilizing hand on the shoulder. The direction of pull should follow the natural arc of the arm as it goes down; this reduces the possibility of destabilizing the patient which would appear to have caused a false weakness in the arm.

4. The doctor can use his own hand to test.

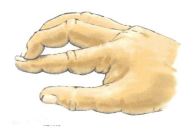

The best way to do this when you are using one hand to locate the points and one hand to test, is to make an arch with the second finger onto the index finger.

When the muscle goes weak the second finger in flexion can override the index finger in extension.

This does take a little practice, so try it enough times before using it with the patient.

One way of practicing this is to talk to yourself (not aloud) and sometimes say something that is true and sometimes something that is false. This could be "I am a man" when you are in fact a woman, or "My name is John" when it is really Michael. Try it and see the difference. It will be good for getting the feel for a weakness.

I have included, below, a few other muscle tests that I have found useful and I hope that you will too.

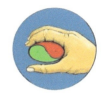

THE ATLAS ROTATION TEST.

This test is useful in cases where it is difficult to palpate the Atlas transverses to determine rotation.

The best way is to have the patient lying supine while the doctor is seated at the patient's head.

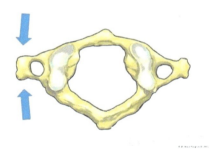

Ask the patient to raise one arm vertically.

Test for a strong arm. In this case the doctor will pull towards himself (cephalic)and the patient will pull towards his feet (caudal).

Place your finger on the posterior margin of the transverse process on the side opposite to the raised testing arm. A light, anterior (towards the ceiling) pressure is sufficient and then test the raised arm. A weakness would indicate an anterior rotation on that side.

Then contact the transverse at the anterior and again press lightly posteriorly. Be careful here as the area just anterior to the transverse is sensitive.

If the arm goes weak then the Atlas has rotated posteriorly on that side.

The transverse has moved in the direction of the challenge.

As an alternative you can just do the posterior contact and anterior pressure on one side and then change sides with both the contact hand and the testing arm and test again.

As you are now using a different arm remember to test again for a strong arm first before making contact with the Atlas.

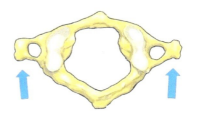

It is easy in this position to retest after the adjustment.

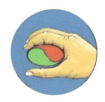

THE SHOULDER TESTS

Occasionally a patient complains of a slight limitation in the movement of the arm. One of the reasons for this can be a slight subluxation of the Humeral Head within the Glenoid Fossa.

This injury can happen from a sudden tug on the arm, or conversely an unprepared brace against a fall etc. The patient feels restriction in a certain movement of the shoulder, sometimes with pain and sometimes without.

These are two tests, to rule out a slight humeral head displacement or subluxation.

Patient is supine. Doctor stands level with the patient's waist, on the side of the shoulder to be tested.

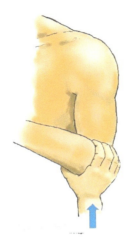

Ask the patient to raise the opposite arm to the vertical position. The doctor reaches across the body to test for a strong arm.

Ask the patient to fully bend the arm to be challenged.

The doctor instructs the patient to completely relax the arm as he contacts the elbow and pushes the humerus, firmly but gently towards the head (cephalic), directly into the shoulder and then tests the opposite arm.

A weakness would indicate a superior subluxation of the humeral head.

TEST TWO

While firmly grasping the arm below the humeral head pull, gently but firmly, down towards the feet (caudal)and again test the opposite arm.

Obviously a weakness would indicate an inferior subluxation of the humeral head.

A weakened arm will indicate that the humeral head has subluxated inferiorly.

Simply put, each test is potentially aggravating the condition, thereby indicating the problem depending on the direction of challenge.

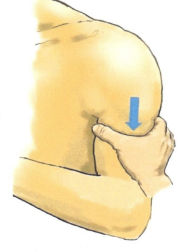

I have had a number of patients with a mysterious and often chronic, slight limitation of shoulder mobility, who have responded immediately following a correction inspired by this test.

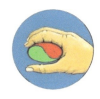

TESTING AN AMPUTEE

What do you do if you have a patient who has had one leg amputated? You still need to determine the **physiological** or **functional** short leg.

The **anatomical** short leg is fairly obvious.

This test applies whether the patient is wearing a prosthesis or not, as it is difficult to accurately test by the normal method in both cases.

I have had a couple of cases of amputees and that is why I came up with this variation, using muscle testing. You can also use this method when you are not sure of the leg lengths on normal testing.

A physiological short leg is a dynamic phenomenon, so if you make a short leg shorter by pushing, or equally making a long leg longer by pulling it, you aggravate the condition and the arm goes weak.

THE AMPUTEE LEG LENGTH TEST.

Either prone or supine, depending on what you are working on, test for a strong arm and then contact one leg and push directly towards the head (Cephalic) then the other one.

The leg that causes the test arm to go weak is the <u>physiological</u> short leg. You can confirm this by pulling one leg at a time down (Caudally) and retest.

Obviously a weakness on one leg would indicate the long leg side. If all is well then the two tests should correlate.

Testing for the long leg. If the arm goes weak then this is the long leg.

Testing for the short leg. If the arm goes weak then this is the short leg.

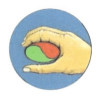

THE FIBULA HEAD TEST.

Persistent lateral knee pain is sometimes caused by a subluxation of the Fibula head on the Tibia. I have come across this on numerous occasions, usually in sportsmen or sportswomen. A sudden twist or perhaps a tackle can cause the Fibula head to displace very slightly, but enough to cause pain.

To determine whether the Fibula has moved anterior or posterior in relationship to the Tibia, a similar muscle test can be done.

When this problem is found by this simple test, the appropriate adjustment can have immediate relief and be most rewarding.

THE FIBULA TEST

The patient is lying supine, with one arm raised perpendicular for testing; the offending knee is bent with the foot on the table, test the testing arm for strength and then contact the posterior surface of the Fibula head and apply an anterior pressure. Test the arm. If it goes weak then the Fibula head has subluxated anteriorly.

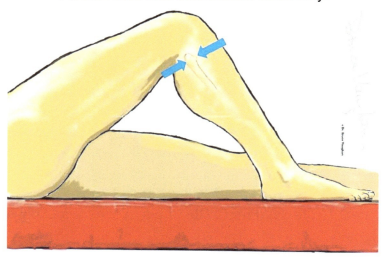

Then contact the anterior surface and apply a Posterior pressure. Test the arm.

If it is weak then the Fibula head has subluxated posteriorly.

Obviously as with most of these tests, if the first test goes weak one has the answer, but it is always a good idea to do both directions to confirm the finding.

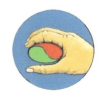

THE HIATAL HERNIA TEST.

I have encountered quite a number of patients who have shown signs of a Hiatal Hernia. This problem can cause them considerable discomfort and sometimes distress, as they are unable to enjoy a meal.

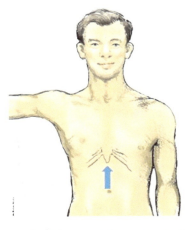

The patient is lying prone with a test arm raised vertically. Test for a strong arm.

The doctor contacts the abdomen with a flat hand, at a point just below the

Use the fingertips of a flat hand to gently but firmly push the stomach up towards the head (cephalic) and then test the arm.

If the arm goes weak this may indicate the presence of a Hiatal Hernia.

I do hope that these tests can be useful for you. I have chosen the ones that I personally use, which can easily become part of your day-to-day routine, without adding much time to the patient visit. They may often save time as they can steer you towards the source of the problem or, in the case of follow-up visits, signs of improvement since the previous visit.

The information that these simple tests can give you is, once you have gained proficiency and have confidence in your testing ability, both valuable and of immediate use.

The time involved is so minimal that there is really no reason why you should not make them part of your routine.

To gain experience I suggest that you do the standing tests on every patient on every visit, regardless of the patient's current complaint, and then do the appropriate prone or supine tests as and where indicated.

There are times when the standing tests, for various reasons, do not seem to indicate a problem, whilst the prone or supine tests do. If you are not convinced by a lack of indicators in the standing tests, especially when you know that there are signs or symptoms indicating a problem, then go to the prone and/or supine tests regardless.

As I have said earlier, do not rely entirely on muscle testing; it is a valuable tool to have in your bag, being a quick and easy way to get information, but with a new patient, or a current patient with a new problem, a thorough examination should of course be done which can, indeed should, include these tests.

Once you gain confidence in your testing, you can be inventive and use the same concept for other articulations.

For a deeper understanding of muscle testing, and of more specific body language testing, as well as a wider use for them, Applied Kinesiology (AK) and Sacro Occipital Techniques (SOT) are definitely worth studying.

About the Author

Dr. Bruce Vaughan DC, FICC,

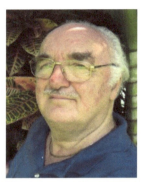

Bruce graduated from Palmer College of Chiropractic in 1966 and has practiced in Hong Kong ever since. He was the founder and President for many years of the Hong Kong Chiropractors Association. Bruce was the first Chairman of the Hong Kong Chiropractors Council.

He served on the World Federation of Chiropractic (WFC) Council for nineteen years, representing Asia and became the President in 2000 – 2002.

Bruce still lives and practices in Hong Kong as the senior partner of Drs. B. S. Vaughan & Associates (Chiropractors). He is the author of five other books and enjoys painting, (the illustrations in this book are all his) travel and gardening. He is also a dog lover.

Books by Bruce Vaughan:
The Basic Approach to SOT
Rabid Dogs in the East
Brazilian Saddle Sores
Regenesis (E-book)
A Matter of Face (E-book)
All are available in Amazon.com and other outlets.

CPSIA information can be obtained
at www.ICGtesting.com
Printed in the USA
LVHW072254260121
677604LV00001B/5